Reflexology for Family and Friends: Simple as 1-2-3

By: Jan Mariette

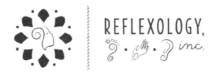

REFLEXOLOGY, inc.

www.reflexologyinc.com

The information presented is not intended or implied to be a substitute for professional medical advice, diagnosis or treatment. All content, including text, graphics, images and information, contained in or available through this book is for general information purposes only. Please see a medical professional if you need help with depression, illness, or have any concerns whatsoever.

Cover and illustrations designed by Lonzo Forester of Gemini Maverick Media™
email: lonzo.forester@inbox.com

ISBN: 978-1500170868

Printed in the United States of America

First and foremost this book is dedicated to my husband, Richard, who has supported and encouraged me in all my endeavors and believed in my ideas often before I did. And secondly to my dear friend and mentor, Bill Hamilton, who is no longer on this earth. Bill gently and lovingly pushed and prodded me and many others at The Garden Retreat to find our true selves and to courageously share our knowledge with the world. My friend and business partner, Donna Lineberger, was my constant cheerleader and proofreader/editor while my friend and yoga instructor, Lisa Gartner, patiently formatted and edited the interior layout to make the book ready for publishing.

Without the help and encouragement of my family and friends I would still just be thinking about writing a book rather than being a published author.

Table of Contents

Reflexology for Family and Friends: Simple as 1-2-3

Introduction

I am a professional reflexologist, certified with over 300 hours of classroom instruction and have owned my own reflexology business for 8 years. I've been the reflexologist at Anderson Cancer Institute in Savannah, Georgia for the past three and a half years as well as a member of their Integrative Health Planning Committee. I love reflexology and I know how beneficial it can be. I've seen firsthand the positive effects it can make in people's lives.

For a few years I had been considering developing a workbook to offer simple training for family or friends, but just never took the steps to follow through. It was because of the positive effects we were noticing with cancer patients and cancer survivors that I began to seriously consider it was time to act. I was only seeing the patients once a week for reflexology sessions at the hospital and I knew I could create a simple instructional program that would allow family members and friends to provide additional sessions between my visits. By having the additional – albeit simplified – routines the patients would experience stress relief and deep relaxation on a more consistent basis. It would also offer family and friend caregivers the opportunity to feel more involved in the positive aspects of the patient's care. Caregivers carry so much of the *have to* issues in the daily lives of any patient, the stress relief/relaxation sessions would be an addition that offers a pleasurable experience to both the patient and the caregiver.

Even though it was the idea of adding an additional layer of positive care for cancer patients that finally motivated me to create this program, the concept is perfect for anyone who is interested in learning how to offer a basic stress relief/deep relaxation session to family or friends. Using the techniques shown is also an excellent addition to your children's bedtime routine helping them to wind down at the end of their day and fall asleep easily.

The instruction included in this book is not a true reflexology course although it does use reflexology techniques. It is a simple program – no anatomy lessons – no specific program for a specific issue – just a very basic, simplified routine that will offer improved blood flow, stress relief, and deep relaxation. It's a program I believe anyone can learn by simply following the directions in the workbook. And who knows, you may be encouraged by this simple instruction to take a full reflexology certification course.

Loving, caring touch offers its own form of comfort and healing. By adding the simple manipulations demonstrated in the material you will be able to offer so much more.

Follow me and let's take the first step on your journey to learning about reflexology!

Jan Mariette
Certified Reflexologist

"Decreasing stress increases your immune cells."
Dr. T. Field, PhD Dir. Touch Research Institute, Univ. of Miami School of Medicine

Reflexology for Family and Friends: Simple as 1-2-3

What is reflexology?

Foot reflexology is the application of pressure to specific points on the feet that will affect corresponding parts of the body. Manipulating specific points on the body to improve health is an ancient practice evidenced in many cultures across 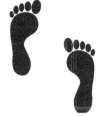 the globe, but modern reflexology as it is known today was developed by two American physicians, Dr. William Fitzgerald of Connecticut and Dr. Joe Shelby Riley of Washington, D.C. around 1913. It was Dr. Riley's assistant, physical therapist, Eunice Ingham, who made reflexology available to the public by teaching family members of patients and then extending her teaching to the general public.

What are some of the benefits of reflexology?
- ❖ Pain management
- ❖ Deep relaxation
- ❖ Improved circulation
- ❖ Stress relief
- ❖ Support during cancer care (pain management, nausea due to chemotherapy, anxiety)
- ❖ Improved quality of sleep

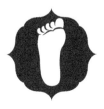

Professional vs. Family and Friends Reflexology Techniques

Professional:

A **_certified_** reflexologist has been educated in anatomy as well as in specific techniques of reflexology and has had a minimum of 200 hours of classroom and practical study of reflexology culminating with written exams and hands-on testing. By knowing and understanding anatomy a certified reflexologist offers a precise, personally specific, reflexology session.

Family and Friends Foot Reflexology:

The manipulations and movements for a basic session are taught without the anatomy study and without the oversight of an instructor. A basic routine can still offer relaxation, stress relief, and improved circulation all of which will also help with pain management.

Although, Reflexology for Family and Friends: Simple as 1-2-3 is not a professional course and cannot be used toward certification it does offer you the skills to help your family and friends feel calm, relaxed, and free from stress.

Enjoy!

What you will need to get started:

- Corn starch
- Pillows
- 2 bath towels
- A comfortable place to work such as a sofa or anti-gravity chair

A small dish or shaker of cornstarch – cornstarch feels silky smooth yet gives you good traction as you are working on the feet. You just need a small amount on your hands and fingers. Place a small amount in the palm of one hand and then rub your hands together as though you are washing them.

Pillows and towels – pillows to place under the feet and behind the back as you are working. You should also place a towel under the feet and one on your lap to prevent getting cornstarch on furniture or clothing.

You will need a comfortable place for the person to sit that gives you easy access to their feet:

- Have them sit on a sofa with their back to one of the arms and their legs stretched out on the seat in front of them with a pillow under their feet. You sit with your back to the opposite arm of the sofa with one of your legs tucked under you and your outer foot resting on the floor. As you begin to work on the feet you may determine that they need to be a bit higher or lower so simply adjust pillows accordingly.
- You could use an anti-gravity lounge chair. If you have one of these they are perfect. Just be sure the foot of your lounge chair raises the feet high enough that you could be in a chair in front of them and their feet would

be above your knees. (These are folding lounge chairs that you can purchase at Bed Bath and Beyond or other stores for approximately $59 or you can buy luxury ones by La Fuma for up to $200. The more expensive ones are lighter weight, but the less expensive ones can still be easily carried.) If you are using an anti-gravity chair place a pillow topped with a towel under the person's feet.

- Some recliners would work, but most do not raise the feet high enough even with pillows under the feet. You want the person's feet to be at a level at or above your navel.

Manipulation Techniques for Reflexology

Before we actually begin a session you will need to know the techniques that are used.

The Inchworm Technique

Inchworm techniques are the movements used most often in a reflexology session.

Thumb inchworm movement

1. Lay the pad of your thumb flat on the skin.

2. Roll your thumb upward by raising your knuckle so that the tip of your thumb is pressing into the skin on the foot of the person receiving reflexology. (Do not press your thumbnail into the skin, just the tip of the thumb.)

3. Then lower your knuckle by sliding your thumb forward.

4. Repeat.

5. You can practice using large movements until you get the feel for it, but when you are actually using the movement in a session the movements are very small, moving forward in the tiniest of increments. (You can see an example by watching the short video on my web site www.reflexologyinc.com)

Index finger inchworm movement

The movement is the same as the thumb, but you are using your index finger as the active tool.

1. Lay the pad of your index finger flat on the skin.

2. Roll your index finger up so that the tip of your finger is pressing the skin of the person receiving reflexology. (Do not press your fingernail into the skin, just the tip of the finger.)

3. Then lower your index finger by sliding it forward to rest the pad on the skin once more.

4. Repeat.

Pressure

Each person has a different threshold for what pressure is best for them, but I can give you an example of where to start.

While seated, place the pad of your thumb very lightly on a flat surface ~ hardly touching the surface at all. Consider that pressure as "1" on a scale of 1-5.

Now, still seated press the pad of the thumb as hard as you can on the flat surface. That would be a "5" on the scale of 1-5.

A good rule of thumb (no pun intended!) would be to start with a pressure of "3" and see how comfortable that is for the person you are working with. The exception to that would be if you are working with infants or the elderly. I use a pressure of "2" with babies and seniors. Seniors can then tell you if they would like more pressure, but babies can't so keep it gentle with babies and toddlers.

Ready?   Let's begin!

Treats

Treats are not reflexology moves, but are meant to get the blood flowing and help to relax the feet. They may also be used to finish each session.

Lightly powder your hands with a small amount of corn starch and you're ready to begin.

Directions for a Basic Reflexology Session – Right Foot

Treat A

With the recipient's right foot resting heel down on the pillow and their foot and toes in an upright position, place your hands on each side of the foot and *roll* the foot briskly back and forth between your hands moving up and down the foot.

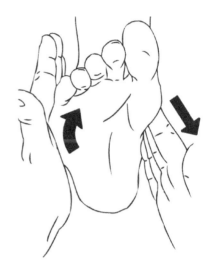

Right – Treat "A"

Treat B

With the recipient's foot in the same position and your hands on both sides of their foot, you rapidly *brush* your hands up and down their foot. When your left hand is down, your right hand is up, alternating quickly in a brushing motion.

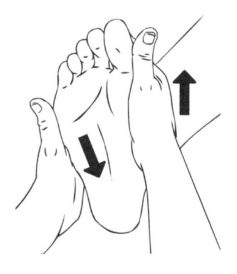

Right – Treat "B"

Treat C

With both of your thumbs on the center of the right sole of the recipient's foot, and with all your fingers on top of their foot, use your fingers to *fold* the top of their foot from the center downward towards you.

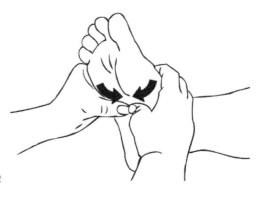

Right – Treat "C"

Treat D

In the same position as in treat "C", keep your fingers on top of their foot and pull and stretch your thumbs outward on their sole. Continue moving upward until you have covered the entire soft sole and ball of foot area.

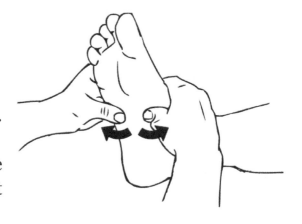

Right – Treat "D"

Top of Right Foot

1. Hold the recipient's right foot in place, upright with their heel on the pillow and your right hand supporting their foot. Use your index finger on your left hand to inchworm down, in the valleys on top of their foot between their toes toward their ankle. Your left thumb is on the sole of their foot. (Right 1)

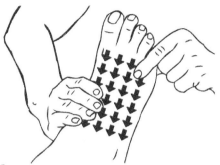

Right 1

2. Do this 2 times in each of the first three valleys.

3. For the fourth valley at their big toe, support their foot with your left hand and use your right index finger to inchworm down the valley 2 times toward their ankle. (No diagram shown)

4. Holding their right foot upright with your left hand, *crawl* the four fingers of your right hand across the top of their upper foot, starting near the inner ankle. (Right 2)

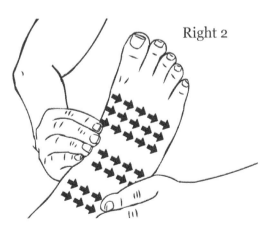

Right 2

5. Then move up and *crawl* your fingers across the mid-section of their upper foot. (Right 6)

6. And then finally *crawl* your fingers across their upper foot near their toes.

7. Next, holding their right foot upright with your right hand, use the four fingers of your left hand to *crawl* across their upper foot once again in all three sections. (Right 3)

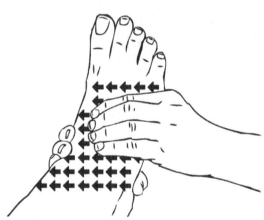

Right 3

Toes of Right Foot

1. Hold their right foot with your right hand. Your left-hand fingers are behind their foot.

2. Beginning with their little toe, use your left thumb to inchworm across the bottom stem of each of their first four toes 2 times. (Right 4)

Right 4

3. Hold their right foot in your left hand and use your right thumb to inchworm across the stem of their big toe from right to left 2 times. (Right 5)

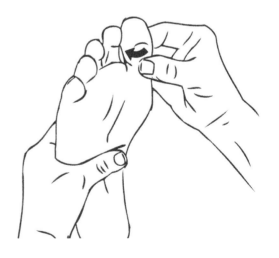

Right 5

4. Hold their right foot upright with your right hand. Your left-hand fingers are behind their foot. (Right 6)

5. Beginning with their little toe, use your left thumb to inchworm across the tips of each toe 2 times (tiny inchworm movements). You will probably need to steady the stem of each toe with your right thumb to keep their toes stable as you inchworm across the top of their toes.

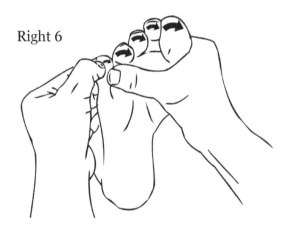

Right 6

6. Hold their right foot upright with your right hand. (Right 7)

7. Use your left thumb to inchworm down the inside of each toe starting with the little toe. Your left thumb will also be pressing each toe down and away from the others as you are working it. Your left fingers will be behind their right toes stabilizing their foot and toes.

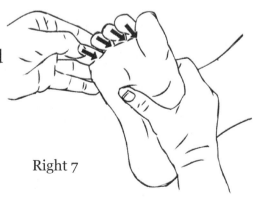

Right 7

8. Now holding the right foot with left hand and using your right thumb begin at the big toe and inchworm down the inside of each toe ending with the toe beside the little toe. (Right 8)

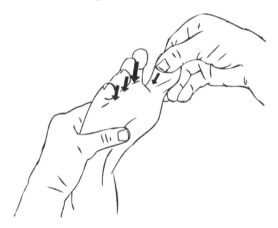

Right 8

9. Holding their right foot with your right hand, use your left fingers to gently *pinch* their little toe from tip to base using very tiny movements Use the pads of your fingers and thumb instead of the tips. (Right 9)

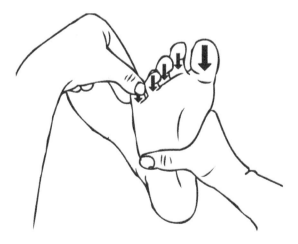

Right 9

10. When you reach the bottom of the little toe, grasp it gently and pull your fingers upwards. Your fingers actually slide up the toe while gently tugging. (No diagram shown)

11. Repeat with the remaining four toes.

12. Hold their right foot with your right hand. Use the pads of your left thumb and index finger to gently pinch the web between the little toe and the toe next to it. Hold for a slow count of 10. (Right 10)

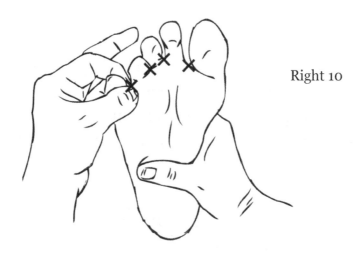

Right 10

13. Do the same for the remaining webs between each of the toes.

Bottom of the Right Foot

1. Continue to hold their right foot with your right hand.

2. Move the fingers of your left hand to a horizontal position behind their right foot.

3. Use your left thumb to inchworm slowly, but deeply, across the line at the base of their toes (where the toes attach to the foot) beginning at the little toe, moving toward the big toe. Your left hand fingers are behind the right foot as a support to allow the thumb to press deeply. Check with the person you are working on to be sure the pressure you are using is deep, but not painful. If it is uncomfortable, use less pressure. You want your recipient to be able to relax and enjoy the session. (Right 11)

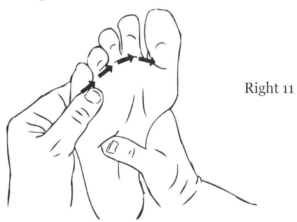

Right 11

4. Inchworm across the foot at the base of the toes at least 2 times.

5. Keep your hands in the same position and move your thumb down slightly in order to inchworm across the upper part of the ball of the foot. (Right 12)

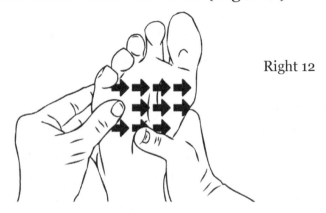

Right 12

6. After the first row, move down lightly, and again inchworm across the foot.

7. Continue moving slightly below the previous line of work until you have covered the entire ball of the foot.

8. Move the fingers of your left hand to a slightly upward diagonal position midway behind their right foot.

9. Use your left thumb to inchworm up the valleys on the ball of the foot. These are the valleys that start at the base of the ball of the foot and move up to between the toes. (Right 13)

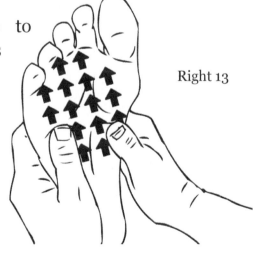

Right 13

10. Start at the valley between the little toe and next toe, inch worming up the valley.

11. Starting at the base of the next valley, inchworm upward.

12. Continue using the same inchworm movement for the remaining 3 valleys.

13. Hold their right foot with your right hand.

14. Place the fingers of your left hand horizontally across the back of their right foot and use your left thumb to inchworm slowly and deeply from left to right across the soft sole just below the ball of the foot. (Right 14)

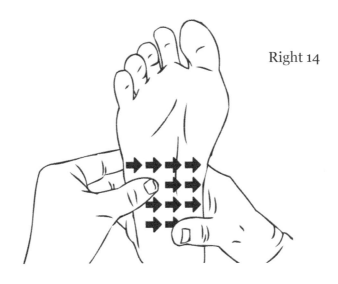

Right 14

15. Once you move completely across the soft sole, go back to the outer edge, move down slightly, and repeat in rows across the soft sole until you reach the heel.

16. Hold the right foot with your left hand. Place the fingers of your right hand behind the right foot.
(Right 15)

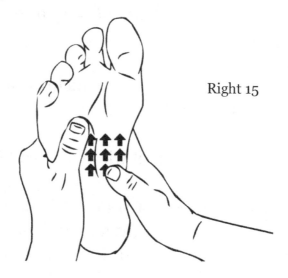

Right 15

17. Your right thumb starts at the base of the soft sole, in line with the big toe, and inchworms in a straight line up to the top of the soft sole.

18. Move your thumb back down to the bottom of the soft sole and slightly to the left of where you just worked and repeat the inchworm up to the top of the soft sole.

19. Continue inchworming up the soft sole until you have covered the entire sole.

20. Repeat at least 2 times.

Right Heel

1. Cup the right heel with your left hand.

2. Wrap the fingers of your right hand across the back of the right foot and use your right thumb to inchworm right to left across the bottom of the heel beginning at the soft sole. (Right 16)

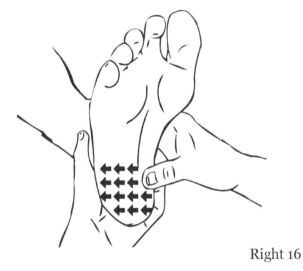

Right 16

3. Continue working across the heel in descending rows until you have covered the entire heel.

4. Repeat 2 times.

Inner Edge of Right Foot

1. Place the fingers of your right hand under the heel of the right foot. (Right 17)

2. Use your left hand to grasp the foot and gently pull to the left.

3. Use your right thumb to slowly and deeply inchworm from the base of the heel up the inner edge of the foot.

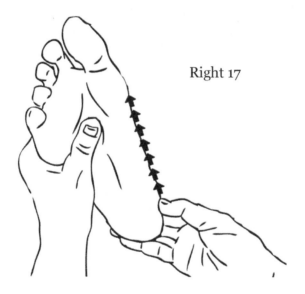

Right 17

4. Stop when you reach the ball of the foot.

5. Repeat 2 times.

Outer Edge of Right Foot

1. Now hold foot with your right hand – fingers on top of foot and thumb below. (Right 18)

2. Pull foot forward and slightly to the right

3. Hold the left hand with the thumb on the outer edge of the foot and right fingers are on the inside edge. (Left palm is facing sole of the foot.)

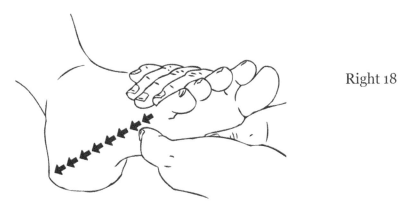

Right 18

4. Using the left thumb inchworm down the outer edge of the foot from the pinkie to the heel. Repeat 2 times.

5. Use your right hand to hold the right foot about mid-foot, and pull gently to the right. (Right 19)

6. Place the fingers of your left hand behind the ankle and use your left thumb to inchworm under the base of the outer ankle.

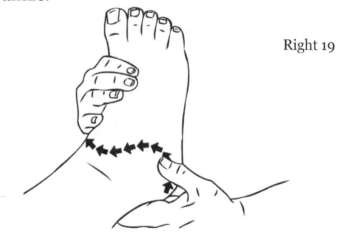

Right 19

7. Gently continue across the top of the ankle. Do this outer ankle/top of ankle movement 2 or 3 times.

Finishing Treats

These are the same as the last two treats described at the beginning.

Treat C

With both of your thumbs on the center of the right sole of the recipient's foot, and with all your fingers on top of their foot, use your fingers to *fold* the top of their foot from the center downward towards you. (Right – Treat C)

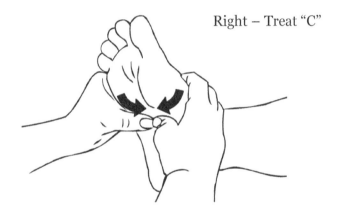

Right – Treat "C"

Treat D

In the same position as in treat "C", keep your fingers on top of their foot and pull and stretch your thumbs outward on their sole. Continue moving upward until you have covered the entire soft sole and ball of foot area. (Right – Treat D)

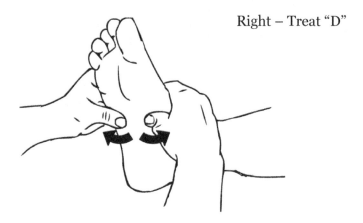

Right – Treat "D"

~NOTES ~

~NOTES ~

Directions for a Basic Reflexology Session – Left Foot

Treat A

With the recipient's left foot resting heel down on the pillow and their foot and toes in an upright position, place your hands on each side of the foot and *roll* the foot briskly back and forth between your hands moving up and down the foot.

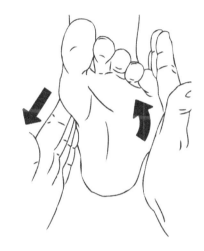

Left – Treat "A"

Treat B

With the recipient's foot in the same position and your hands on both sides of their foot, you rapidly *brush* your hands up and down their foot. When your left hand is down, your right hand is up, alternating quickly in a brushing motion.

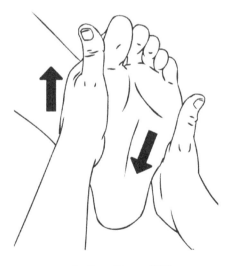

Left – Treat "B"

Treat C

With both of your thumbs on the center of the left sole of the recipient's foot, and with all your fingers on top of their foot, use your fingers to *fold* the top of their foot from the center downward towards you.

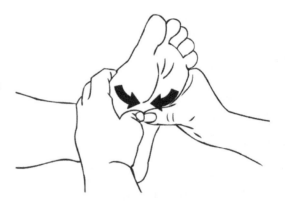

Left – Treat "C"

Treat D

In the same position as in treat "C", keep your fingers on top of their foot and pull and stretch your thumbs outward on their sole. Continue moving upward until you have covered the entire soft sole and ball of foot area.

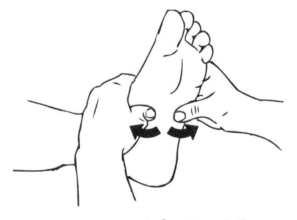

Left – Treat "D"

Top of Left Foot

1. Hold the recipient's left foot in place, upright with their heel on the pillow and your left hand supporting their foot. Use your index finger on your right hand to inchworm down, in the valleys on top of their foot between their toes toward their ankle. Your right thumb is on the sole of their foot. (Left 1)

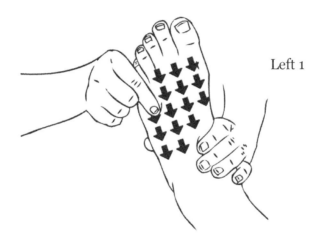

Left 1

2. Do this 2 times in each of the first three valleys.

3. For the fourth valley at their big toe, support their foot with your right hand and use your left index finger to inchworm down the valley 2 times toward their ankle. (No diagram shown)

4. Holding their left foot upright with your right hand, *crawl* the four fingers of your left hand across the top of the foot, starting near the ankle. (Left 2)

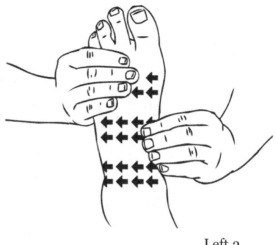

Left 2

5. Then *crawl* your fingers across the mid-section of their upper foot.

6. And then finally *crawl* your fingers across their upper foot near their toes.

7. Next, holding their left foot upright with your left hand, use the four fingers of your right hand to *crawl* across their upper foot once again in all three sections. (Left 3)

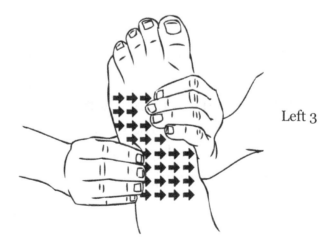

Left 3

Toes of Left Foot

1. Hold their left foot with your left hand. Your right-hand fingers are behind their foot. (Left 4)

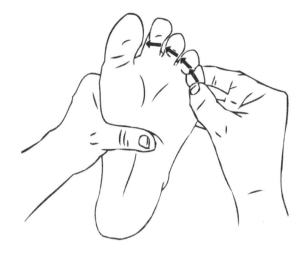

Left 4

2. Beginning with their little toe, use your right thumb to inchworm across the bottom stem of each of their first four toes 2 times.

3. Hold their left foot in your right hand and use your left thumb to inchworm across the stem of their big toe from left to right. Repeat 2-3 times. (Left 5)

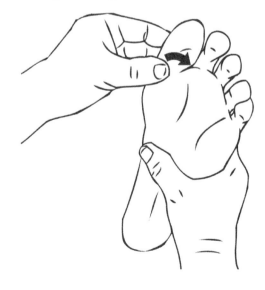

Left 5

4. Hold their left foot upright with your left hand. Your right-hand fingers are behind their foot. (Left 6)

5. Beginning with their little toe, use your right thumb to inchworm across the tips of their toes 2 times. You will probably need to steady the stem of each toe with your left thumb to keep their toes stable as you inchworm across the tops.

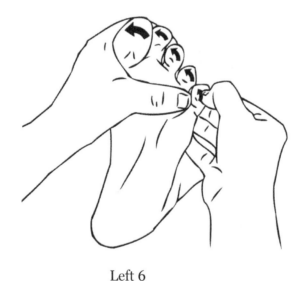

Left 6

6. Hold their left foot upright with your left hand. (Left 7)

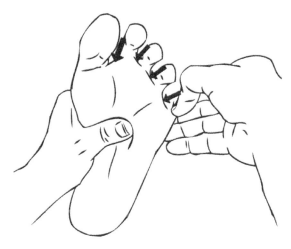

Left 7

7. Use your right thumb to inchworm down the inside of each toe starting with the little toe. Your thumb will also be pressing each toe down and away from the others as you are working it. Your right fingers will be behind their right toes stabilizing their foot and toes.

8. Now hold left foot upright with your right hand and using your left thumb begin with their big toe and inchworm down the inside of each toe ending with the toe next to the little toe. (Left 8)

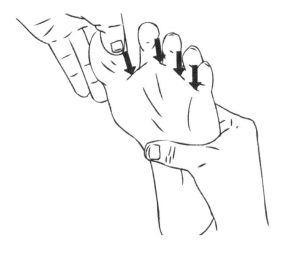

Left 8

9. Holding their left foot with your left hand, use your right fingers to gently *pinch* their little toe from tip to base. Use the pads of your fingers and thumb instead of the tips. (Left 9)

10. When you reach the bottom of the little toe, grasp it gently and pull your fingers upwards. Your fingers actually slide up the toe while gently tugging. (No diagram shown)

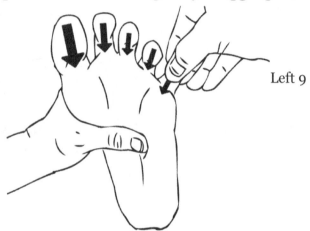

Left 9

11. Repeat with the remaining four toes.

12. Hold their left foot with your left hand. Use your right thumb and index finger to gently pinch the web between the little toe and the toe next to it. Hold for a slow count of 10. (Left 10)

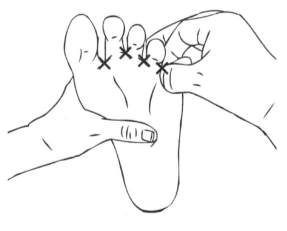

13. Do the same for the remaining webs between each of the toes.

Bottom of the Left Foot

1. Continue to hold their left foot with your left hand.

2. Move the fingers of your right hand to a horizontal position behind their left foot. (Left 11)

3. Use your right thumb to inchworm slowly, but deeply, across the line at the base of their toes (where the toes attach to the foot) beginning at the little toe moving toward the big toe. Your right hand fingers are behind the left foot as a support to allow the thumb to press deeply. Check with the person you are working on to be sure the pressure you are using is deep, but not painful. If it is uncomfortable, use less pressure. You want your recipient to be able to relax and enjoy the session.

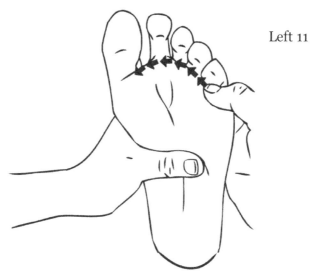

Left 11

4. Inchworm across the foot at the base of the toes at least 2 times.

5. Keep your hands in the same position and move your thumb down slightly in order to inchworm across the upper part of the ball of the foot. (Left 12)

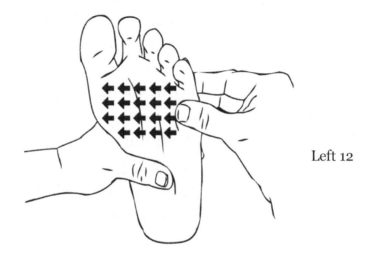

Left 12

6. After the first row, move down slightly, and again inchworm across the foot.

7. Continue moving slightly below the previous line of work until you have covered the entire ball of the foot.

8. Move the fingers of your right hand to a slightly upward diagonal position midway behind their left foot. (Left 13)

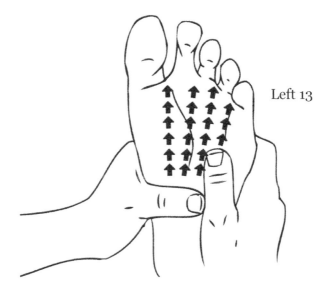

Left 13

9. Use your right thumb to inchworm up the valleys on the ball of the foot. These are the valleys that start at the base of the ball of the foot and move up to between the toes.

10. Start at the valley between the little toe and next toe, inch-worming up the valley.

11. Starting at the base of the next valley, inchworm upward.

12. Continue using the same inchworm movement for the remaining 3 valleys.

13. Hold their left foot with your right hand. (Left 14)

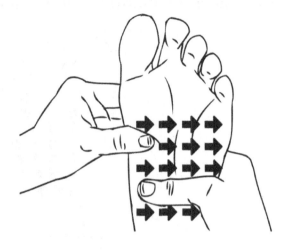

Left 14

14. Place the fingers of your left hand horizontally across the back of their left foot and use your left thumb to inchworm slowly and deeply from left to right across the soft sole just below the ball of the foot.

15. Once you move completely across the soft sole, go back to the inner edge, move down slightly, and repeat in rows across the soft sole until you reach the heel.

16. Hold the left foot with your right hand. Place the fingers of your left hand behind the left foot. (Left 15)

17. Your left thumb starts at the base of the soft sole, in line with the big toe, and inchworms in a straight line up to the top of the soft sole.

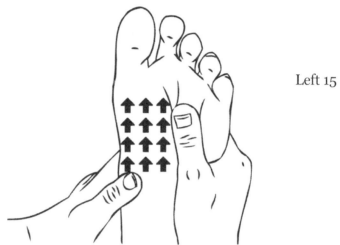

Left 15

18. Move your thumb back down to the bottom of the soft sole and slightly to the right of where you just worked and repeat the inchworm up to the top of the soft sole.

19. Continue inch worming up the soft sole until you have covered the entire sole.

20. Repeat at least 2 times.

Left Heel

1. Cup the left heel with your right hand.
2. Wrap the fingers of your left hand across the back of the left foot and use your left thumb to inchworm left to right across the bottom of the heel beginning at the soft sole.

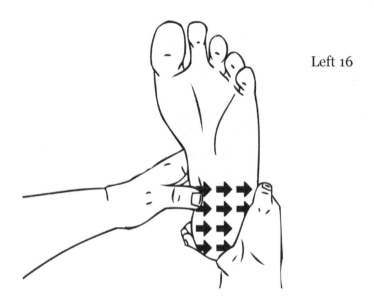

Left 16

3. Continue working across the heel in descending rows until you have covered the entire heel.

4. Repeat 2 times.

Inner Edge of Left Foot

1. Place the fingers of your left hand under the heel of the left foot. (Left 17)

2. Use your right hand to grasp the foot and gently pull to the right.

3. Use your left thumb to slowly and deeply inchworm from the base of the heel up the inner edge of the foot.

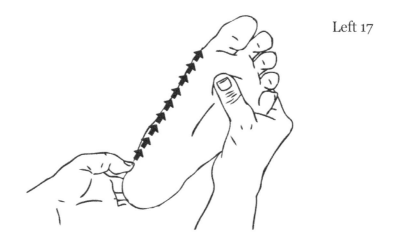

Left 17

4. Stop when you reach the ball of the foot. Repeat 2 times.

Outer Edge of Left Foot

1. Now hold foot with your left hand – fingers on top of foot and thumb below. (Left 18)

2. Pull foot forward and slightly to the left.

3. Hold the right hand with the thumb on the outer edge of the foot and right fingers are on the inside edge. (Right palm is facing the sole of the foot.)

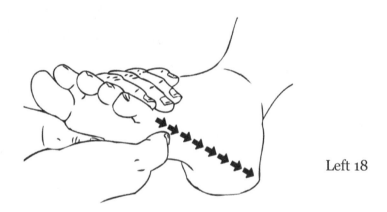

Left 18

4. Using the right thumb inchworm down the outer edge of the foot from the pinkie to the heel. Repeat 2 times.

5. Using your left hand, hold the left foot about mid-foot, and pull gently to the left. (Left 19)

6. Place the fingers of your right hand behind the ankle and use your right thumb to inchworm under the base of the outer ankle.

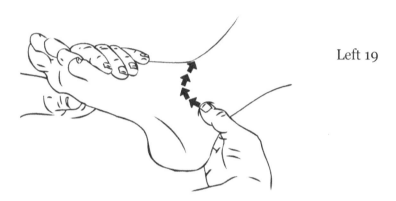

Left 19

7. Gently continue across the top of the ankle. Do this outer ankle/top of ankle movement 3 or 4 times.

Finishing Treats

These are the same as the first two treats described in the beginning.

Treat C

With both of your thumbs on the center of the left sole of the recipient's foot, and with all your fingers on top of their foot, use your fingers to *fold* the top of their foot from the center downward towards you.

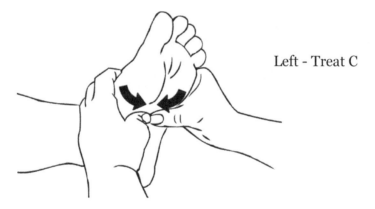

Left - Treat C

Treat D

In the same position as in treat "C", keep your fingers on top of their foot and pull and stretch your thumbs outward on their sole. Continue moving upward until you have covered the entire soft sole and ball of foot area.

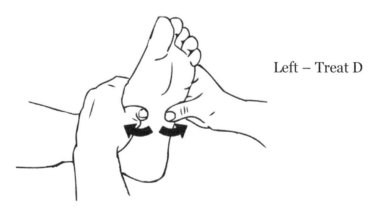

Left – Treat D

~NOTES ~

~NOTES ~

PLEASE consider sharing your book with a friend so that the two of you can work with one another. You deserve a deep relaxation session as well!

Right Foot Illustrations

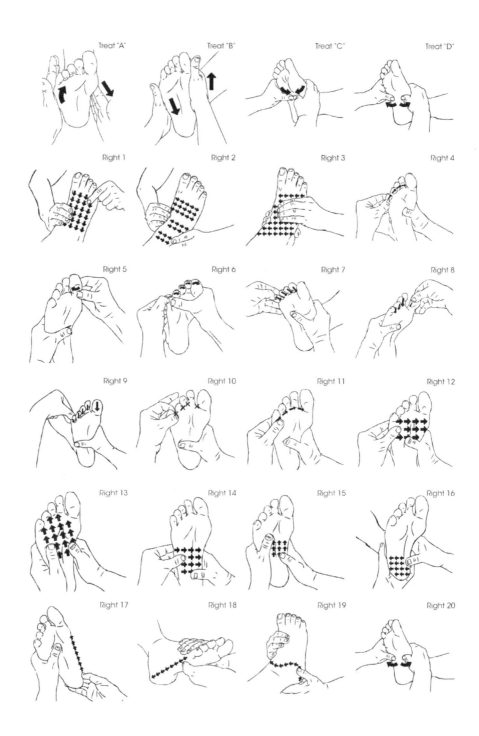

Left Foot Illustrations

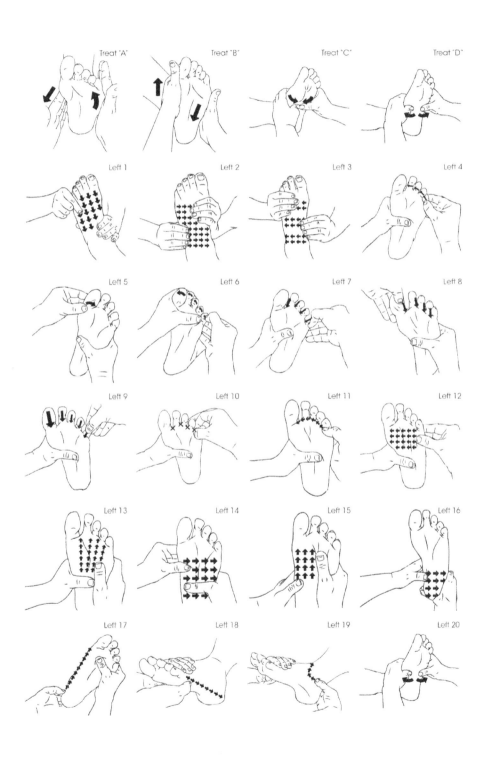

ABOUT THE AUTHOR

Jan Mariette is a Reflexologist and Reiki Master/Teacher, certified in Feet, Hand and Ear Reflexology through the American Academy of Reflexology and in Facial Reflexology through the Instituto de Reflexologia (Sorensensistem).

She owns and operates Reflexology, Inc. in Savannah, Georgia, where she is also the reflexologist at Memorial University Medical Center's Anderson Cancer Institute and is a member of their Integrative Health Planning Committee.

Ms. Mariette lives in coastal Georgia where she and her husband share their home with a cat and three rescue dogs. She is currently working on the next book in her "Simple as 1-2-3" series.

Made in the USA
Las Vegas, NV
12 April 2024

88537898R00037